Copyright 2023

Table of Contents

Lupus is a disease that occurs when your body's immune system attacks your own tissues and organs (autoimmune disease). Inflammation caused by lupus can affect many different body systems — including your joints, skin, kidneys, blood cells, brain, heart and lungs.

Lupus can be difficult to diagnose because its signs and symptoms often mimic those of other ailments. The most distinctive sign of lupus — a facial rash that resembles the wings of a butterfly unfolding across both cheeks — occurs in many but not all cases of lupus.

Some people are born with a tendency toward developing lupus, which may be triggered by infections, certain drugs or even sunlight. While there's no cure for lupus, treatments can help control symptoms.

BREAKFAST

1. French Baked Toast with Cream and Eggs

Prep Time: 5 Minutes

Cook Time: 15 Minutes

Servings: 2

Ingredients

- 2 tablespoons salted butter, softened
- 2 pieces thick sliced bread such as brioche
- ½ cup heavy cream
- 1 clove garlic, thinly sliced
- 1 bay leaf
- salt and pepper to taste
- 4 large eggs
- 2 teaspoons chopped fresh chives

Instructions

1. Preheat the oven to to 375 degrees.

2. Butter each piece of bread on both sides using one tablespoon for each.

3. Heat a large oven proof skillet over medium-high heat then add the bread. Cook until toasted and golden, turn, then cook until golden on the other side. Repeat with the other slice of bread, then arrange the bread slices side by side in the pan.

4. Add the cream to a small saucepan along with the garlic and bay leaf, then bring to a simmer over medium-low heat. Season to taste with salt and pepper and let simmer for about 5 minutes. Remove the bay leaf and the garlic if you're sensitive (I prefer to leave it in). Pour two tablespoons of hot cream over each slice of bread.

5. Carefully crack two eggs over each piece of bread, being very careful not to break the yolks. Pour the remaining cream over the eggs, then transfer to the center rack of the oven.

6. Bake until the whites are just set but the yolks are still runny, about 13 minutes.

7. Sprinkle with chives and more freshly ground pepper if desired. Serve immediately.

Prep Time: 5 Minutes

Cook Time: 20 Minutes

Servings: 4

Ingredients

- 1/2 cup grated Parmesan cheese
- 1/2 cup crème fraîche
- 2 tablespoons fresh parsley, chopped
- salt and pepper to taste
- 1 sheet store-bought Puff Pastry, thawed
- 1 egg, beaten
- 5 slices cooked bacon
- 4 eggs, divided
- 1 cup arugula, watercress, or microgreens
- red pepper flakes (optional)

Instructions

1. Preheat oven to 400 degrees F and line a half-sheet baking pan with parchment.

2. Mix Parmesan cheese, créme Fraiche, and chopped fresh parsley in a small bowl. Season with salt, pepper; set aside.

3. On a lightly floured surface, roll out thawed puff pastry sheet into a large rectangle that fits on the baking sheet. Score the puff pastry with a knife to create a 1-inch border. Dock the interior puff pastry rectangle with a fork. Then brush the border edges with one beaten egg. Refrigerate dough for 10 minutes to create maximum rise.

4. Spread the créme Fraiche mixture in the center of the pastry. Place bacon strips or chopped bacon over the cheese mixture. Bake for 15-20 minutes or until the pastry is puffed and golden brown and the bacon is cooked through. Remove from the oven.

5. Poach the eggs: While the pastry tart is baking, poach the eggs. Here's a post on how we poach eggs.

6. Remove the tart from the oven, season with salt and pepper to taste, and an optional sprinkling of red pepper flakes. Top with poached eggs and garnish with arugula, watercress, or microgreens. Serve immediately.

Prep Time: 15 Minutes

Cook Time: 15 Minutes

Servings: 8

Ingredients

- 2 cups all-purpose flour
- 4 teaspoons baking powder
- 1 tablespoon pure honey
- 3/4 teaspoon salt
- 1/3 cup cold butter, diced
- 1/2 cup shredded cheddar (Scottish or your preference)
- 1/4 cup chopped green onions (1 to 2 scallions, small chop)
- 3/4 cup milk
- 1 egg for egg wash
- freshly ground black pepper
- Ham, spinach or arugula, whole-grain mustard, and fried eggs to serve

Instructions

1. Preheat the oven to 450 degrees F and line a baking sheet with parchment.

2. In a large bowl or the bowl of a food processor, mix flour, baking powder, sugar, and salt. Using a pastry blender, fork, or the metal blade of a food processor, cut in the butter until the mixture is crumbly. Stir in shredded cheese, green onions, and milk, just until the dry ingredients are moistened.

3. Drop dough onto parchment lined or ungreased baking sheet by 8 to 12 spoonfuls, about 2 inches apart. Brush with beaten egg, sprinkle with a dusting of freshly ground black pepper and bake 12 to 15 minutes or until golden brown.

4. Slice the biscuits in half and serve with ham, spinach or arugula, whole grain mustard and fried eggs.

Prep Time: 20 Minutes

Cook Time: 20 Minutes

Servings: 10-12

Ingredients

For The Zucchini Fritters:

- 1 pound (about 2 medium) zucchini
- 1 teaspoon plus ½ teaspoon salt, divided
- ¼ cup chopped chives or scallions (green parts only)
- 1 large egg
- Freshly cracked black pepper, to taste
- ½ cup all-purpose flour
- 1 tablespoon corn starch
- ½ teaspoon baking powder
- Oil, for frying

For The Lemon Herb Yogurt Sauce (Optional):

- 1 cup plain, full-fat Greek yogurt or sour cream
- 1 small clove of garlic, minced or grated with a microplane grater
- 2 tablespoons fresh lemon juice

- ¼ teaspoon salt
- freshly cracked black pepper, to taste
- 2 tablespoons chopped chives or scallions (green parts only)
- 2 tablespoons chopped assorted fresh herbs (basil, lemon thyme, dill, tarragon, parsley, chervil, etc.)

Instructions

1. Grate the zucchini using either the grating attachment on a food processor or the large holes on a box grater.
2. Sprinkle the zucchini with 1 teaspoon of salt, gently mix, then spread out onto a large kitchen towel and let sit for about 20 minutes to release its liquid.
3. Fold up the towel and wring it our over a bowl or sink to extract the liquid. Be aggressive and really squeeze out as much liquid as your can.
4. In a medium bowl, mix together the chives or scallions, egg, flour, corn starch, baking powder, pepper and the remaining ½ teaspoon of salt.
5. Add the zucchini and mix until everything is thoroughly combined.

6. Heat about a ¼ - ½ inch of oil in a large skillet over medium-high heat, then line a baking sheet with paper towels and set it aside nearby.

7. Carefully drop heaping spoonfuls of the zucchini mixture into the hot oil and lightly press with the back of the spoon to flatten. Be careful not to overcrowd the pan. About 4 per batch is usually just right.

8. Cook until the edges are golden, about 3 to 4 minutes. Flip the fritters and fry them on the other side for another 2-3 minutes, until nicely browned, then remove to the paper towels to drain.

9. To make the sauce, add the yogurt, garlic, lemon juice, salt, pepper, chives or scallions and herbs in a small bowl and mix to combine. Taste, and adjust the seasoning as needed.

10. Serve the fritters while they're hot with the lemon herb yogurt on the side.

11. To serve later, place the fritters in a 200 degree F oven until ready to serve.

Prep Time: 10 Minutes

Cook Time: 45 Minutes

Servings: 10-12

Ingredients

- 8–10 cups cubed bread
- 2 cups cooked and cubed ham
- 2 cups shredded cheese (I used an Italian mix)
- 9 large eggs
- 2 cups milk (dairy or non-dairy works)
- 1 teaspoon salt
- 1 teaspoon ground mustard
- 1/4 teaspoon fresh ground black pepper, plus more for topping
- 3 green onions, chopped

Instructions

1. Generously grease a 9×13 inch casserole dish or spray with nonstick spray.

2. Layer in the bread, ham, and green onions. Then sprinkle cheese evenly over the top.

3. In a large bowl, whisk together the eggs, milk, salt, ground mustard, and pepper. Pour evenly over the bread in the casserole dish. Top with additional green onions and pepper is desired.

4. Cover tightly and refrigerate for 2 hours to 12 hours (or overnight).

5. When ready to bake, remove the strata from the refrigerator and let sit out while the oven preheats to 375 degrees F.

6. Bake casserole, uncovered, for 30 minutes. Then loosely cover with foil or parchment for the remaining 20 to 25 minutes. The strata is done with the edges are nicely browned the center is puffy.

7. Remove from the oven and let cool for a few minutes before serving.

Prep Time: 10 Minutes

Cook Time: 20 Minutes

Servings: 2-4

Ingredients

For The Croutons:

- 3 cups torn or cubed day-old cornbread (homemade or store bought)
- 1 tablespoon olive oil
- salt and freshly cracked black pepper

For The Dressing:

- 2 anchovies packed in oil
- 2 cloves garlic, minced
- salt and freshly cracked black pepper
- 2 teaspoons Dijon mustard
- 2-3 tablespoons freshly squeezed lemon juice
- ½ teaspoon Worcestershire sauce
- 2 tablespoons mayonnaise
- 2 tablespoons vegetable oil

For The Salad:

- 1 large bunch kale, any variety, ribs removed and torn into pieces
- 2 teaspoons extra virgin olive oil
- salt and freshly cracked black pepper
- ½ cup finely grated parmesan cheese, plus more for garnish

Instructions

Make The Croutons

1. Line a baking sheet with parchment paper and preheat the oven to 350 degrees. Toss the cornbread with olive oil, salt and pepper, then spread out evenly on the baking sheet. Bake for about 20 minutes, checking on them occasionally, or until they're golden brown and crisp. Allow to cool to room temperature. Store in an air tight container for up to one week.

Make The Dressing

1. Place the anchovies and garlic in a bowl, sprinkle with salt and pepper, then use the back of a spoon to grind the mixture into a paste. Add the mustard, the lemon juice and Worcestershire sauce and whisk to combine.

Add the mayonnaise and vegetable oil and whisk until emulsified. Taste and adjust seasoning as needed, adding more salt, pepper and lemon juice to suit your preference.

Make The Salad

1. Place the kale in a large salad bowl and drizzle with oil, salt and pepper. Use clean hands to vigorously massage the leaves until they wilt and soften, about 2 minutes. Drizzle with desired amount of dressing and toss until all the leaves are coated. Sprinkle with parmesan cheese and continue tossing until evenly distributed. Add a few handful of croutons and toss some more. Spoon into serving bowls, top with more cheese and croutons if desired. Serve immediately.

Prep Time: 20 Minutes

Cook Time: 10 Minutes

Servings: 2

Ingredients

- 1 small clove garlic, finely grated on a microplane
- juice of 1 lemon
- ¼ cup tahini
- kosher salt, to taste
- cold water, as needed
- 1 large head cauliflower, leaves and stem trimmed
- freshly ground pepper, to taste
- 4 tablespoons olive oil, divided
- flaky sea salt, such as Maldon, for sprinkling
- 2 tablespoons pine nuts, toasted
- ¼ cup pomegranate arils
- ¼ cup fresh cilantro or mint leaves, torn

Instructions

2. Combine the garlic, lemon, tahini and salt in a bowl. Whisk together and add cold water, a tablespoon at a time while whisking. The mixture will seize up at first. Keep whisking and adding water until it forms a smooth, saucy consistency. Taste for seasoning and adjust with more lemon and salt as needed.

3. Place the cauliflower stalk-side-down on a cutting board and trim ¼ off the edge on either side. Cut two thick slices (about 1 ½-2 inches) out of the middle, then save the remaining crumbled edge pieces for another use (like soup or a salad).

4. Preheat the oven to 350 degrees and place a sheet pan inside to heat up. Heat 3 tablespoons olive oil in a large cast iron skillet over high heat. Season the cauliflower steaks on both sides with salt and pepper, then carefully place one in the hot pan. Reduce the heat to medium-high and let cook until dark brown, about 5 minutes. Carefully flip and cook until dark brown on the other side. Transfer to the oven, then pour the remaining tablespoon of olive oil in the pan and repeat with the remaining cauliflower steak. The steaks are done when a knife can easily pierce the middle of each.

5. Spoon a generous amount of tahini sauce on each plate, then place the cauliflower steaks on top. Sprinkle with flaky sea salt, then scatter the pomegranate arils and pine nuts all around. Garnish with a few cilantro or mint leaves, and serve immediately.

Prep Time: 10 Minutes

Cook Time: 30 Minutes

Servings: 4

Ingredients

- 1 tablespoon olive oil
- 8 bone-in, skin-on chicken thighs (about 3 lbs)
- salt and pepper
- 6-8 oil-packed anchovies
- 3 garlic cloves, smashed*
- 2 sprigs fresh rosemary*
- 2 tablespoons white wine vinegar
- ½ cup dry white wine
- ¼ cup water

Instructions

1. Heat olive oil in a large dutch oven or wide, heavy-bottomed pot or pan with high sides over medium-high heat.

2. Season chicken thighs all over with salt and pepper, then place 4 of them in the pan skin-side-down and cook until browned, about 5 minutes. Flip and cook until browned on the other side, about 5 minutes more, then transfer to a plate and repeat with the remaining chicken thighs.

3. Lower the heat, then add the anchovies to the pan and stir until they start to break down and dissolve in the fat. Add the garlic and rosemary and sauté for about a minute.

4. Deglaze the pan with vinegar, white wine and water, then nestle the chicken pieces back into the pan. Bring the sauce up to a boil, then reduce the heat to keep it at a low simmer. Spoon some of the sauce over each chicken thigh, then cover and cook for about 20 minutes, or until the chicken is fully cooked and tender.

5. Remove the lid and allow the sauce to reduce and thicken for about 10 minutes more.

6. Remove the rosemary sprigs and garlic cloves if desired, then serve.

Prep Time: 5 Minutes

Cook Time: 25 Minutes

Servings: 6

Ingredients

- 5 slices bacon, diced
- 1 shallot, sliced
- 4 cups (loosely packed) raw kale, hard stems removed
- 2 cups cooked and cubed butternut squash
- 8 eggs
- ¾ teaspoon salt
- black pepper to taste
- 4 oz goat cheese

Instructions

1. Preheat the oven to 400 degrees.
2. Place the bacon in a cold, heavy bottomed, oven safe pan (cast iron is ideal), and bring up to medium heat. Render the bacon until it's just beginning to crisp, abut 5 minutes. Add the shallot to the pan and cook

for 2-3 minutes, until its translucent and just starting to brown. Add the kale to the pan with a splash of water, and toss it around for a few minutes, then throw a lid on the pan and let it steam for 2-3 minutes, or until tender. Remove the lid and add the cooked squash, then toss around until it's warmed through.

3. Crack the eggs into a medium bowl, add the salt and pepper, and whisk until thoroughly combined. Pour the eggs over the vegetables and use a rubber spatula to spread them out evenly. Crumble the goat cheese over the top, then place the pan in the oven for 10-15 minutes, until puffed up and golden on the outside. The inside should be totally set. If it's still runny, place back in the oven for a few minutes more.

4. Allow the frittata to rest for 5-10 minutes before slicing. Serve warm or at room temperature.

Prep Time: 1hrs 5 Minutes

Cook Time: 25 Minutes

Servings: 16

Ingredients

- 2 ½ cups all purpose flour
- ¼ cup stoneground cornmeal
- 2 tablespoons sugar
- 1 scant teaspoon salt
- ½ cup plus 6 tablespoons (1 ¾ sticks) cold unsalted butter, cut into small cubes
- ¼ cup vegetable shortening, I prefer nonhydrogenated
- 1 large egg yolk, white reserved
- 2 tablespoons (or more) ice water

For The Filling

- 2 cups hulled strawberries, sliced
- 2 tablespoons sugar
- 1 tablespoon corn starch
- pinch of salt

- 6 ounces goat cheese

- 2 tablespoons lemon thyme leaves, optional

- flaky sea salt for sprinkling, optional

Instructions

To Make The Dough

1. Combine the flour, cornmeal sugar and salt in a bowl
   and whisk together. Use a pastry cutter or your fingers
   to cut the butter and shortening into the flour until
   they become pieces the size of peas.

2. Add in the egg yolk and water, adding more one
   tablespoon at a time until the dough JUST comes
   together. Be very careful not to overmix the dough. As
   soon as it comes together, don't knead it any further.

3. Divide the dough in two, form it into rectangular
   pieces, wrap and chill in the refrigerator for at least 30
   minutes and up to over night.

Make The Filling

1. While the dough is chilling, prepare the filling.
   Combine the strawberries, sugar, corn starch and salt
   in a medium sauce pan. Bring up to a boil, then

reduce to a simmer, and cook until thick, about 5 minutes. Set aside and allow to cool.

Assemble The Tarts

1. Roll out each rectangle of dough on a lightly floured surface to about 14" wide and 18" long. Trim the excess to square off any uneven edges and then cut 16 even rectangles out of each - 4 long x 4 wide.

2. Divide the goat cheese evenly among half of the squares, then top with a heaping tablespoon of strawberry filling. Sprinkle each with the lemon thyme, reserving some for the tops.

3. Cut a vent in the remaining 16 rectangles. I used the back of a pastry tip to make a little hole, but you can use a knife or small cookie cutters.

4. Whisk the reserved egg white with a teaspoon of water until it's broken up. Working one at a time, brush the edges of each vented rectangle and place over top of the filling. Press down on the edges, then use the tines of a fork to make sure each pastry is fully sealed. Place on a parchment lined baking sheet (you will need two or more to make all 16) and repeat with the rest.

5. When all pastries are finished, place the sheet pans in the freezer while you preheat the oven to 425 degrees. When the oven is preheated, remove the pans and

brush with the remaining egg white and top with a light sprinkling of flaky sea salt and more lemon thyme.

6. Bake for about 25 minutes, or until golden brown. Allow to cool for at least 10 minutes before serving. Be careful - the filling will be very hot.

11. Cherry Vanilla Ricotta Crostata

Prep Time: 30 Minutes

Cook Time: 1hrs 15 Minutes

Servings: 6-8

Ingredients

For The Crust

- 1 cup flour
- 1 teaspoon salt
- 1 teaspoon sugar
- 4 tablespoons very cold butter
- 2 tablespoons vegetable shortening (I prefer non hydrogenated)
- 5 tablespoons ice water

For The Filling

- 1 cup full fat ricotta cheese
- ¼ cup, plus 2 tablespoons sugar, divided
- 1 vanilla bean, split lengthwise and seeds scraped

- 2 pints fresh cherries, pitted (about 3 heaping cups of fruit)
- pinch of salt
- 1 egg beaten
- 1 tablespoon sugar in the raw (optional)

Instructions

For The Crust

1. Combine the flour, salt and sugar in a medium bowl. Use a pastry cutter to cut in the butter and shortening until the pieces become the size of peas. Add in 6 tablespoons of water and mix gently with a rubber spatula or wooden spoon until the dough just starts to come together. Add more water one tablespoon at a time if needed. The dough should not be sticky, and you should be able to see the pieces of butter and shortening flecked throughout. Be careful not to over knead it.

2. Form dough into a roughly shaped rectangle, wrap in plastic and refrigerate for at last 30 minutes (or up to two days).

Make The Filling

1. In a medium bowl, combine the ricotta cheese with ¼ cup sugar, half of the vanilla seeds and set

2. aside. In another bowl, mix together the pitted cherries, 2 tablespoons of sugar, the remaining vanilla seeds and a tiny pinch of salt.

Assemble The Tart

1. Preheat the oven to 375 degrees. Remove the dough from the fridge and roll it out to an oval/rectangle roughly 16" x 10" in size - it doesn't have to be perfect, this is a rustic tart. Roll up the dough on to the rolling pin and transfer it to a large baking sheet that's been lined with parchment paper.

2. Spread the ricotta mixture on the dough in an even layer, leaving a 2-3" border around the edges. Arrange the cherries evenly on top of the ricotta and pour over any juice. Gather the edges and fold them up around the mixture to hold everything in.

3. Brush the edges with the beaten egg, then sprinkle with raw sugar if desired. Place in the oven and cook for about 30 minutes or until the edges are golden brown. Remove from the oven and allow to cool. Serve warm, at room temperature, or cold. Store any leftovers in the refrigerator for up to 5 days.

Prep Time: 10 Minutes

Cook Time: 25 Minutes

Servings: 8

Ingredients

- 2 tablespoons olive oil
- 1 onion medium, chopped
- 3 cloves garlic minced
- 2 teaspoons ground cumin
- 2-3 teaspoons chili powder
- 1 teaspoon dried oregano
- 1 teaspoon fine sea salt
- freshly ground black pepper to taste
- pinch of red pepper flakes (optional)
- 4 cups cubed squash (like pumpkin or butternut squash)
- 1 bell pepper medium, chopped
- 3 small to medium zucchini, chopped (about 2 cups)
- 1 (15-ounce) can tomatoes, diced with liquid (fire-roasted is nice)
- 1 (15-ounce) can pinto beans, drained and rinsed

- 1 (15-ounce) can red kidney beans, drained and rinsed
- 2 cups corn kernels fresh or frozen
- 3 to 4 cups water
- ¼ cup fresh cilantro or parsley, fresh, chopped

Instructions

1. Heat the olive oil in a soup pot or Dutch oven. Add the chopped onion and sauté over medium-low heat until softened and beginning to caramelize; 3 to 5 minutes. Stir in the garlic, cumin, chili powder, oregano, salt, pepper, and red pepper flakes if using; continue to sauté until the spices are fragrant, about 30 seconds.
2. Add the cubed squash, bell pepper, zucchini, tomatoes, and drained beans to the pot. Pour in 3 cups of water and bring to a simmer.
3. Cover and gently simmer until the vegetables are tender; 20 to 25 minutes. Add additional water if needed. The stew should be thick and moist, but not overly soupy. It will continue to thicken as it cools.
4. Season with salt and pepper to taste. Before serving, garnish with fresh cilantro or parsley.

Prep Time: 15 Minutes

Cook Time: 1hrs 12 Minutes

Servings: 8

Ingredients

Equipment

- Dutch Oven
- 2 Tbsp olive oil
- 2 cups onion chopped (about 1 medium)
- 2 cups carrots peeled and chopped
- 2 garlic cloves minced
- 2 tsp ground cumin
- 1 cup dried lentils rinsed
- 4 cups vegetable broth (or chicken broth)
- 2 cups water
- 1 15-ounce canned diced tomatoes
- 1 tbsp brown sugar
- 1 cinnamon stick
- 1/2 cup dry barley

- 3 cups Swiss chard chopped (or other green like kale or spinach)
- salt and pepper to taste

Instructions

1. Heat oil over medium heat in a Dutch oven and add onion and carrots; cook until the vegetables begin to soften. Add garlic and cumin and cook for another minute.
2. Stir in lentils, broth, tomatoes, brown sugar and cinnamon stick; bring the soup to a boil.
3. Reduce the heat to maintain a simmer and add barley. Cover and cook for about 60 minutes, or until the barley is tender.
4. Stir in the chard, cover, and cook until tender; about 5 minutes. Add parsley and season with salt and pepper to taste before serving.

Prep Time: 10 Minutes

Cook Time: 30 Minutes

Servings: 2

Ingredients

Equipment

- Nonstick Stovetop Grill
- 2 4-ounce salmon filets
- 1 tablespoon olive oil extra virgin
- salt and pepper to taste
- 2 cups sweet potatoes roasted
- 4 cups salad greens (spinach, kale, arugula, etc)
- 1 avocado chopped
- 2 ounces walnuts (roasted, salted or candied)
- 1/2 cup blueberries
- Lemon Vinaigrette
- 1/4 cup lemon juice
- 1 garlic minced
- 1 tsp Dijon mustard
- 1/2 tsp honey

- 1/3 cup olive oil extra virgin
- 1/2 tsp dried thyme
- salt and pepper to taste

Instructions

1. Make the Lemon Vinaigrette by whisking the ingredients together and store in a lidded jar in the refrigerator. This step can be done in advance.

2. To roast the sweet potatoes: Preheat the oven to 400°F. Chop the sweet potato into cubes and toss in 1 to 2 tablespoons of olive oil. Spread on a baking sheet and season with salt and pepper. Roast for 30 minutes. This step can be done in advance and refrigerated until ready to make the salad.

3. To grill the salmon: Season with salt and pepper and heat oil in a large skillet or grill over medium-high heat. Place salmon on the grill, skin side up, for 4 minutes, or until the flesh begins to brown. Carefully turn and cook until it's done, about 4 to 5 minutes more.

4. In a salad bowl, toss the greens with the sweet potatoes. Top the salad with salmon, avocado, blueberries, and walnuts. Drizzle with lemon

vinaigrette just before serving. Season with salt and pepper to taste.

15. Hungarian Mushroom Soup

Prep Time: 15 Minutes

Cook Time: 35 Minutes

Servings: 6

Ingredients

- Dutch Oven
- Hungarian Sweet Paprika
- 4 tablespoons unsalted butter
- 2 cups onions chopped
- 2 garlic cloves minced
- 1 pound mushrooms sliced
- 2 cups vegetable broth or chicken broth
- 1 tablespoon soy sauce
- 1 tablespoon paprika sweet Hungarian style
- 2 teaspoons dried dill
- 1 cup milk
- 3 tablespoons all-purpose flour
- 1/4 cup sour cream or plain yogurt
- 3 tablespoons fresh parsley chopped
- 2 teaspoons lemon juice
- 1 teaspoon salt

- black pepper to taste

Instructions

1. Melt butter or olive oil in a large pot over medium heat. Add onions and mushrooms; sauté until softened, about 10 minutes. Stir in garlic and cook 1 minute more.
2. Stir in broth, soy sauce, paprika, and dill; reduce heat to low, cover, and simmer for 15 minutes.
3. Whisk milk and flour together in a separate bowl; stir into soup until blended. Cover and simmer for 15 more minutes, stirring occasionally.
4. Add sour cream (or yogurt), fresh parsley, lemon juice, salt, and ground black pepper; stir over low heat until warmed through.

16. One Pot Pumpkin Mac and Cheese

Prep Time: 15 Minutes

Cook Time: 15 Minutes

Servings: 6-8

Ingredients

- 2 tablespoons butter
- 3 cloves garlic, minced or pressed
- 1 tsp dried thyme
- 1 pound pasta (macaroni, shells, etc.)
- 1 cup milk (dairy or non-dairy, I used coconut milk)
- 3 ounces cream cheese
- 1 (15-ounce) canned pumpkin puree
- 1½ cups shredded sharp cheddar cheese
- 1 teaspoon onion powder
- 1 teaspoon paprika
- 1/4 teaspoon cayenne pepper
- 1/4 teaspoon nutmeg
- salt and pepper to taste

Instructions

1. Melt butter in a large pot or Dutch oven over medium heat. Once the butter has melted add the minced garlic and dried thyme; sauté for about 30 seconds.

2. To the pot, add the pasta and toss in the butter garlic mixture. Add 4 cups of water and bring to a boil over high heat. Add 1 1/2 teaspoons salt and cooking, stirring occasionally for 8 to 9 minutes. Without draining the water, stir in the milk, cream cheese, and pumpkin; cook until the cream cheese has melted and the pasta is al dente.

3. Remove the garlic and stir in the shredded cheese, onion powder, paprika, turmeric, cayenne, and nutmeg until the cheese has melted and the pasta is creamy. Remove from the heat.

4. Season with salt and pepper to taste and add up to 1/4 cup water or milk to thin the pasta if necessary.

Prep Time: 15 Minutes

Cook Time: 30 Minutes

Servings: 4-6

Ingredients

- 1 tablespoon olive oil
- 1 medium onion, chopped
- 2 carrots, chopped
- 2 ribs celery, chopped
- 2 green bell peppers, chopped
- 1 jalapeno pepper, chopped (optional for added heat)
- 3 cloves garlic, chopped
- 2 tablespoons chili powder
- 1 teaspoon ground cumin
- 1 1/2 teaspoons smoked paprika
- 1 teaspoon dried oregano
- 1 teaspoon salt
- 2 (15 ounces) cans diced tomatoes with juices
- 2 (15 ounces) cans black beans, rinsed and drained
- 1 (15 ounces) can pinto beans, rinsed and drained
- 2 cups water

- 1 bay leaf

Instructions

1. Heat the olive oil in a large Dutch oven over medium heat. Add chopped onions, bell peppers, jalapeno (if using), carrots, and celery. Season with a pinch of salt and cook, stirring occasionally until the vegetables are softening, and the onion is translucent; about 5 to 7 minutes.

2. Stir in the garlic, chili powder, cumin, smoked paprika, and oregano and cook until fragrant; about 1 minute.

3. Add the tomatoes with their juices, black and pinto beans, water, and bay leaf. Stir to combine and bring the chili to a simmer. Maintain a simmer and cook, stirring as needed, for 30 minutes.

4. Remove from the heat and stir in fresh parsley or cilantro, season to taste with salt and pepper, and serve with favorite toppings. Squeeze a bit of lime into chili before serving for a pleasing balance of acidity.

Prep Time: 10 Minutes

Cook Time: 10 Minutes

Servings: 6-8

Ingredients

- 1 1/2 cups uncooked orzo
- 3/4 cup crumbled feta
- 1/4 cup red onion chopped
- 1 (10 ounce) package cherry tomatoes, halved
- 1 English cucumber, chopped
- 1/4 cup Greek olives, pitted and halved
- 1/4 cup fresh parsley, chopped
- Vinaigrette
- 1/2 cup olive oil
- 1 garlic clove, minced or pressed
- 1/4 cup red wine vinegar
- 2 teaspoons honey
- 1/2 teaspoon dried oregano
- Pinch red pepper flakes (optional for heat)
- Salt & pepper to taste

Instructions

1. Cook orzo al dente according to package directions; for about 7 minutes. Drain and rinse with cold water.

2. Make the Vinaigrette

3. Combine the garlic, red wine vinegar, honey, oregano, and red pepper flakes if using in a blender. With the blender running, gradually blend in the olive oil. Season with salt and pepper to taste. This vinaigrette keeps well in the refrigerator for 3 to 4 days.

4. Assemble the Greek Orzo Salad

5. In a large bowl, add feta, red onion, tomatoes, cucumber, and olives. Add the cooled orzo and drizzle in the vinaigrette. Toss to coat and season with additional salt and pepper to taste. Fold in the fresh parsley and chill until ready to serve.

Prep Time: 15 Minutes

Cook Time: 30 Minutes

Servings: 6-8

Ingredients

- 1 teaspoon olive oil
- 6 to 8 boneless skinless chicken thighs
- 4 slices of bacon, chopped into 1/4-inch pieces
- 1 onion, chopped
- 3 cloves garlic, minced
- 1 green bell pepper, chopped
- 2 cups white rice (long or medium grain)
- 3/4 cup cherry tomatoes
- 2 (15-ounce) cans chicken broth
- 1 bay leaf
- 1 teaspoon salt
- 1/2 teaspoon black pepper
- pinch of red pepper flakes
- 1/4 cup chopped fresh parsley for garnish

Instructions

1. Preheat the oven to 325 degrees F.

2. Heat olive oil in a large heavy-bottomed pot or Dutch Oven. Season the chicken with salt and pepper and brown on all sides. Remove the chicken from the pan and transfer to a plate; set aside.

3. Reduce heat to medium and add the bacon. Cook until browned; about 4 minutes. Stir in the onion and green pepper; saute until softened and translucent. Stir in the garlic and cook for 1 minute more. Finally, stir in the rice until it's coated.

4. To the pot, add the tomatoes, chicken stock, 1 cup water, bay leaf, and red pepper flakes (if using). Bring to a simmer, stirring well, then add the chicken thighs and bring back to a simmer.

5. Cover and bake in the oven for 30 minutes. To serve, garnish with fresh parsley.

Prep Time: 15 Minutes

Cook Time: 30 Minutes

Servings: 6-8

Ingredients

- 3/4 lb meat in bite-size portions (flank steak, rotisserie chicken, or tofu)
- 1 tablespoon canola oil
- 3–4 cup chopped vegetables (I love to use peppers, spinach, baby bok choy, onions, broccoli or buy pre-chopped in your produce section).
- cilantro as garnish

Stir Fry Sauce:

- 1/4 cup soy sauce
- 3 tablespoons brown sugar
- 1/4 cup water
- 2 tablespoons white vinegar
- 2 garlic cloves, minced
- 1/2 teaspoon freshly grated ginger
- 1 teaspoon sriracha, or to taste

Instructions

1. Stir Fry Sauce: Make the sauce by adding all of the ingredients into a mason jar, secure with lid, and shake. Set aside.

2. Make rice or noodles to serve with stir fry.

3. Meat: If using uncooked meat, cut into bite size pieces, add to a skillet coated with canola oil and heated over medium-high heat. Stir fry until done. Transfer to a bowl and set aside. If using rotisserie chicken, stir fry until heated through and set aside.

4. Veggies: In the same skillet, add canola oil and chopped veggies. Stir Fry over medium-high heat until crisp-tender.

5. Add the meat back into the skillet and about half of the stir fry sauce, or to taste. Swirl until meat and veggies are coated and hot. Serve over rice or noodles.

21. Minestra Maritata (Italian Wedding Soup)

Prep Time: 20 Minutes

Cook Time: 20 Minutes

Servings: 6

Ingredients

- 4 tablespoons extra-virgin olive oil, divided
- 1 ⅓ cups chopped yellow onion
- ⅔ cup chopped carrot
- ⅔ cup chopped celery
- 2 tablespoons minced garlic
- 6 cups unsalted chicken broth
- 6 ounces orzo, preferably whole-wheat
- 1 ½ tablespoons chopped fresh oregano
- ½ teaspoon kosher salt
- 24 cooked chicken meatballs (12 ounces), such as Easy Chicken Meatballs (see associated recipe)
- 4 cups baby spinach
- ¼ cup grated Parmesan cheese

Instructions

1. Heat 1 tablespoon oil in a large pot over medium-high heat. Add onion, carrot, celery and garlic; cook, stirring occasionally, until the onion is translucent, 4 to 5 minutes.
2. Add broth, cover and bring to a boil. Add orzo, oregano and salt; cover and cook, stirring occasionally, until the orzo is just tender, about 9 minutes.
3. Stir in meatballs and spinach; cook until the meatballs are heated through and the spinach is wilted, 2 to 4 minutes.
4. Serve sprinkled with cheese and drizzled with the remaining 3 tablespoons oil.

Prep Time: 10 Minutes

Cook Time: 20 Minutes

Servings: 4

Ingredients

- Large skillet
- Saucepan
- Mixing bowls
- ¼ cup extra-virgin olive oil
- 2 Tbsp. fresh lemon juice
- 2 cloves garlic, minced
- 1 tsp. smoked paprika
- 1 tsp. dried oregano
- ¾ tsp. kosher salt
- ½ tsp. black pepper
- 1 lb. raw peeled and deveined shrimp
- 2 small zucchinis, sliced into coins
- 2 bell peppers (color of choice), sliced into 1x1" pieces
- 1 cup dry farro or white rice
- 2 cups vegetable or chicken broth
- Optional garnishes:

fresh herbs, cherry tomatoes, sliced green olives or capers

- Lemon-Garlic Yogurt
- ½ cup plain whole-milk Greek yogurt
- 1 garlic clove, grated (I use a microplane) sub 1 tsp. granulated garlic
- 1 Tbsp. lemon juice
- ¼ tsp. kosher salt

Instructions

1. In a small bowl, combine first seven ingredients (olive oil through black pepper); stir with a whisk. Place shrimp and vegetables in two separate bowls, and divide marinade evenly into each one; toss to coat. Let stand 5 to 10 minutes.

2. Meanwhile, combine farro or rice in a saucepan with broth. Bring to a boil, reduce heat to low, and gently simmer, covered, until grains are tender and most liquid is absorbed. (This will take about 15 minutes for white rice, and up to 30 minutes for farro.)

3. Meanwhile, heat a large skillet coated in cooking spray (or lightly greased with oil) over medium-high. Once hot, add shrimp and cook 2 minutes per side, or until opaque. Transfer to a plate. (If your skillet isn't

large enough to fit all shrimp in a single layer, cook in two batches.) Next, add vegetables to the same skillet and cook until tender, about 8 minutes.

4. Prepare Lemon-Garlic Yogurt by combining yogurt, garlic, lemon juice, and salt in a small bowl. Stir in 1 to 2 Tbsp. water to thin out to desired consistency.

5. Assemble bowls by dividing farro or rice evenly into each of 4 bowls. Scatter shrimp and vegetables overtop, and finish with a dollop of Lemon-Garlic Yogurt. If desired, garnish with sliced cherry tomatoes, olives, or fresh herbs. Finish with a drizzle of olive oil.

Prep Time: 15 Minutes

Cook Time: 2hrs 20 Minutes

Servings: 6

Ingredients

- 1 lb ground turkey
- 1 tablespoon olive oil
- 1 medium onion, chopped finely
- 1 green bell pepper, chopped finely
- 1 red bell pepper, chopped finely
- 3 cloves garlic, crushed
- 2 teaspoons ground cumin
- 2 teaspoons chili powder
- 3/4 cup quinoa, rinsed
- 1 cup salsa
- 2 1/2 cups chicken stock
- 2 cans (15-ounces) black beans, drained and rinsed
- 1 cup corn kernals (fresh, frozen, or canned)
- 1/2 cup fresh cilantro sprigs

Instructions

1. Heat oil in a large skillet over medium-high heat. Add ground turkey and saute, breaking it up as it cooks; about 3 minutes. Stir in onions, peppers, and garlic and cook until the vegetables begin to soften; 2 to 3 minutes. Add the chili powder and ground cumin to the skillet and cook for 1 minute more. Transfer to a 6-quart slow cooker.

2. Add the rinsed quinoa, salsa, stock, and black beans to the slow cooker; stir to combine. Cover and cook on low for 2 hours and 30 minutes. One hour before the chili has finished cooking, add the corn and cook until tender. Season to taste.

3. Top quinoa chili with cilantro sprigs, lime, and sour cream if desired.

Prep Time: 15 Minutes

Cook Time: 35 Minutes

Servings: 4

Ingredients

- 1 large sheet pan
- 1 lb. small to medium Yukon Gold or red potatoes, halved or quartered, depending on size
- 4 (6-oz.) skin-on salmon fillets
- 3 Tbsp. extra-virgin olive oil (or avocado oil), divided
- 1 tsp. chili powder
- 1 tsp. granulated garlic
- 1 ¼ tsp. kosher salt, divided
- ½ tsp. black pepper, divided
- 1 (8-oz.) pkg. French green beans (haricots verts), trimmed
- Zest of 1 lemon (reserve juice for Garlic Herb Sauce)

Garlic Herb Sauce:

- ¼ cup sour cream or mayonnaise
- 1 Tbsp. fresh lemon juice

- 1 Tbsp. chopped fresh parsley plus more for garnish
- 2 tsp. Dijon mustard
- 1 tsp. minced garlic sub ½ tsp. granulated garlic
- Dash of salt and black pepper

Instructions

1. Preheat oven to 425°F. Arrange potatoes, cut side down, on a large rimmed baking sheet, spacing evenly apart. Add 1 ¼ cups water (just enough to coat the baking sheet), and place in the oven. Bake for ~25 minutes, until the potatoes are fork-tender and water has evaporated. (Note: if any water remains, blot it with a kitchen towel or carefully drain in the sink.)

2. While the potatoes bake, begin preparing salmon. Pat salmon dry with a paper towel, and brush 1 Tbsp. of the oil evenly over flesh and skin. In a small bowl, combine chili powder, garlic powder, and ½ tsp. salt. Sprinkle seasoning mixture evenly over salmon flesh, and let stand 5 to 10 minutes.

3. Push potatoes to one half of the baking sheet and toss with 1 ½ Tbsp. oil, ½ tsp. salt, and ¼ tsp. black pepper. Arrange salmon fillets in the center of the

baking sheet, and transfer back to the oven. Bake for 5 minutes.

4. Add green beans to the open side of the pan, and toss with remaining ½ Tbsp. oil, ¼ tsp. salt, and ½ tsp. black pepper. Place pan back in the oven and bake for 10 minutes. Turn on broiler to high; broil until salmon is golden, about 2 minutes.

5. During the final bake, prepare Garlic Herb Sauce by combining sour cream (or mayo), lemon juice, parsley, Dijon mustard, and garlic in a small bowl. Stir with a whisk, and season to taste with salt and pepper. Stir in 1 to 2 tsp. water to thin out to desired consistency.

6. Garnish salmon with lemon zest, and potatoes with additional chopped fresh parsley, if desired. Serve with lemon wedges and Garlic Herb Sauce.

Prep Time: 20 Minutes

Cook Time: 15 Minutes

Servings: 6

Ingredients

- Large skillet
- Mixing bowls
- ¾ cup pecan halves
- 6 to 8 oz. halloumi cheese
- 2 to 3 Tbsp. corn starch
- 2 Tbsp. extra-virgin olive oil
- 2 ripe fuyu persimmons
- 1 (5-oz.) bag or container baby arugula
- 2 roasted and peeled red beets, sliced into segments (optional) (I use the pre-roasted, vacuum-sealed beets sold in the produce section, such as Love Beets brand)
- 1 medium avocado, sliced

White Wine Vinaigrette:

- 2 Tbsp. minced shallots

- 2 Tbsp. white wine vinegar (sub sherry vinegar or champagne vinegar)
- 1 tsp. honey
- 1 tsp. Dijon mustard
- ½ cup extra-virgin olive oil
- ½ tsp. each sea salt and cracked black pepper

Instructions

Prepare White Wine Vinaigrette:

1. In a glass jar with a fitted lid (or large liquid measuring cup), combine all dressing ingredients. Shake or mix well until combined. Set aside.
2. Toast pecans one of two ways (trust me, this step is worth it!):
3. In the Oven: Preheat oven to 325°F. Arrange pecans in a single layer on a baking sheet. Toast until browned and fragrant, shaking the pan occasionally, about 7 to 10 minutes.
4. On the Stove: Toast pecans in a medium skillet over medium heat until fragrant, stirring occasionally, about 3 to 5 minutes.

5. You'll know the pecans are toasted when they smell like pecan pie! Let cool for 5 minutes before roughly chopping.

Prepare Halloumi Croutons:

1. Cut halloumi into small cubes and toss in a bowl with corn starch until well-coated.

2. Heat 2 Tbsp. olive oil in a large skillet over medium-high. Once the oil is shimmering, arrange halloumi in pan. Cook until halloumi is golden and crispy, only flipping every 1 to 2 minutes to allow each side to sear. Transfer to a paper towel-lined plate.

3. Lay each persimmon on its side and slice off the stem. Cut thin, crosswise slices, and then cut each slice into quarters (refer to photo in text for reference).

4. Place arugula in a large bowl or serving platter and toss with half of the dressing. Arrange persimmons, beets, avocado, toasted pecans, and halloumi croutons overtop. Pour remaining dressing evenly overtop.

Prep Time: 20 Minutes

Cook Time: 55 Minutes

Servings: 4

Ingredients

- Baking sheet
- Large skillet with fitted lid
- 2 medium acorn squashes
- 3 Tbsp. extra-virgin olive oil divided
- ¾ tsp. kosher salt, divided
- 8 oz. sliced baby bella (cremini) mushrooms
- ½ cup finely chopped shallots
- 2 cloves garlic minced
- 6 thyme sprigs
- ½ cup dry quinoa
- 1 cup vegetable broth
- ¾ cup whole milk (sub unsweetened cashew milk)
- ¼ tsp. black pepper
- 6 Tbsp. grated parmesan cheese divided
- 2 to 3 Tbsp. balsamic glaze (homemade or store-bought)

- Pomegranate arils for garnish (optional)

Instructions

1. Preheat the oven to 425°F and line a large, rimmed baking sheet with parchment paper or foil for easy clean-up.

2. Cut acorn squash in half, lengthwise; scoop out seeds and discard. Brush flesh evenly with 2 Tbsp. olive oil and season evenly with ½ tsp. salt. Place flesh side-down on baking sheet. Bake until the squash flesh is easily pierced through by a fork, about 30 minutes. Leave the oven on.

3. Meanwhile, heat remaining 1 Tbsp. oil in a large skillet (with a fitted lid) over medium-high. Add mushrooms and shallots; cook 6 to 8 minutes, until soft. Add garlic; cook 1 more minute. Stir in quinoa and cook for 1 to 2 minutes, to lightly toast grains.

4. Stir in broth, milk, remaining ¼ tsp. salt, and black pepper. Add thyme sprigs and bring mixture to a simmer. Cover, reduce heat to low, and cook until quinoa absorbs liquid and is fluffy; about 17 to 20 minutes.

5. Remove lid and stir in 3 Tbsp. of the Parmesan cheese. Remove thyme sprigs.

6. Fill the hollow center of each squash half with quinoa mixture. Sprinkle remaining parmesan cheese overtop. Place back in the oven for 10 to 15 more minutes, until the tops are lightly golden.

7. Remove from oven and drizzle balsamic glaze over squash halves. Garnish with pomegranate arils. Enjoy right out of the skin!

Prep Time: 20 Minutes

Cook Time: 20 Minutes

Servings: 4

Ingredients

- Large skillet
- Mixing bowls
- 1 ¼ lbs. center-cut salmon, skin removed
- ¾ tsp. kosher salt, divided
- 4 Tbsp. extra-virgin olive oil, divided
- 1 Tbsp. honey
- 2 tsp. gochujang (Korean red pepper paste)
- 3 Tbsp. white sesame seeds
- 3 Tbsp. black sesame seeds
- 1 crown broccoli, cut into florets (about 6 cups total)
- ¼ tsp. black pepper
- Cooked long-grain white rice for serving
- Kimchi and thinly sliced green onion for garnish (optional)

Creamy Miso-Ginger Sauce:

- 1 Tbsp. white miso paste
- 2 Tbsp. seasoned rice vinegar
- 2 Tbsp. toasted sesame oil
- 2 Tbsp. mayonnaise (I use avocado oil mayo)
- 1 tsp. minced fresh ginger
- ½ tsp. gochujang (Korean red pepper paste)
- ½ tsp. honey

Instructions

1. Cut salmon into 1x1-inch cubes and season evenly with ½ tsp. salt.
2. In a large bowl, combine 2 Tbsp. of the olive oil, honey, and gochujang; whisk to combine. Add salmon and gently turn to coat.
3. Combine sesame seeds on a large plate or wide-rimmed shallow bowl, mixing to disburse colors. Add salmon cubes and turn to coat in sesame seeds.
4. Prepare Creamy Miso-Ginger Sauce: In a medium bowl, combine miso and vinegar; whisk to combine. Add sesame oil, mayonnaise, ginger, gochujang, and honey; mix until smooth. Set aside.
5. Heat 1 Tbsp. olive oil in a large skillet over medium-high. Once hot, add broccoli florets. Cook 7 to 8

minutes, tossing occasionally, until crisp-tender. Season with remaining ¼ tsp. salt and black pepper, and transfer to a bowl. Cover to keep warm.

6. Add remaining 1 Tbsp. oil to hot pan. Arrange salmon cubes in a single layer and let cook, undisturbed, for 2 minutes. Stir, and continue cooking for 3 to 5 more minutes, turning to sear all sides, until nicely golden.

7. Serve salmon and broccoli on top of a bed of white rice. Garnish with a spoonful of kimchi, and drizzle Miso-Ginger Sauce over everything. If desired, garnish with thinly sliced green onion.

Prep Time: 20 Minutes

Cook Time: 30 Minutes

Servings: 6

Ingredients

- Small saucepan
- Baking sheet
- Mixing bowls
- 4 heaping cups peeled and cubed butternut squash
- 2 Tbsp. extra-virgin olive oil
- ½ tsp. salt, divided
- 1 cup dry quinoa
- 2 cups vegetable broth
- 2 packed cups kale, stemmed and roughly chopped (lacinato or green curly kale)
- 1 ½ cups shredded red/purple cabbage
- 1 cup matchstick carrots
- 1 red bell pepper, thinly sliced (optional)
- ⅓ cup roasted peanuts, roughly chopped
- 3 Tbsp. fresh chopped basil leaves
- 1 avocado, peeled and sliced or cubed (optional)

Creamy Ginger Dressing:

- 2 Tbsp. tahini (or peanut butter)
- 2 Tbsp. lime juice
- 2 Tbsp. sweet red chili sauce (I use Thai Kitchen brand)
- 1 Tbsp. honey or maple syrup
- 2 tsp. fish sauce (or soy sauce)
- ½ tsp. freshly grated ginger
- ¼ tsp. kosher salt
- ¼ cup extra-virgin olive oil

Instructions

1. Preheat oven to 400°F. Toss squash in 2 Tbsp. oil ¼ tsp. salt; spread evenly on a rimmed baking sheet. Place in the oven and bake for 25 to 35 minutes, tossing once halfway through, until the squash is tender and lightly browned.
2. Meanwhile, combine quinoa and broth in a small saucepan. Bring mixture to a boil, cover, reduce heat, and gently simmer until liquid is absorbed and quinoa is fluffy, about 15 minutes. Transfer to a large bowl.

3. Prepare Creamy Ginger Dressing by combining all ingredients except olive oil in a small bowl; stir to combine. Gently stream in olive oil, whisking constantly, until dressing is smooth.

4. Add kale to bowl with quinoa, and toss to combine (the residual heat of the quinoa will help soften the kale leaves). Add cabbage, carrots, bell pepper (if using), and butternut squash. Season with remaining ¼ tsp. salt. Add dressing and gently toss to combine. Stir in peanuts and fresh basil, and garnish with avocado (if using).

Prep Time: 20 Minutes

Cook Time: 20 Minutes

Servings: 4

Ingredients

- Large skillet with fitted lid
- 2 Tbsp. extra-virgin olive oil
- 1 cup diced yellow onion
- 1 pint cherry tomatoes, halved
- 8 oz. dry penne pasta
- 1 cup marinara sauce
- 2 cups water
- ½ tsp. garlic powder
- ½ tsp. dried oregano
- ½ tsp. each kosher salt and cracked black pepper
- 2 to 3 generous handfuls fresh baby spinach
- ⅓ cup heavy cream
- ½ cup shredded mozzarella cheese
- ¼ cup chopped fresh basil leaves
- Grated Parmesan cheese for garnish (optional)

Instructions

1. Heat 2 Tbsp. oil in a large skillet with a fitted lid over medium heat. Add onion and tomatoes; cook 7 to 8 minutes, until the onion is soft and tomatoes are broken down and jammy.

2. Add pasta, marinara sauce, water, garlic powder, oregano, salt, and pepper. Increase heat to medium-high and bring mixture to a simmer. Cover and cook, stirring occasionally, until the pasta is al dente, 10 to 12 minutes.

3. Remove lid and stir in heavy cream, spinach, and cheese. Stir continuously until spinach wilts and cheese melts, about 2 minutes. Garnish with fresh basil and Parmesan, if using.

Prep Time: 15 Minutes

Cook Time: 45 Minutes

Servings: 4

Ingredients

- Large pot
- Rimmed baking sheet
- Mixing bowls
- 3 garlic cloves, unpeeled
- ¼ cup plus 1 tsp. extra-virgin olive oil, divided
- 1.5lbs. baby yellow potatoes
- 2 Tbsp. finely chopped fresh rosemary
- 1 Tbsp. ground sumac
- 2 ½ tsp. kosher salt, divided
- ½ tsp. cracked black pepper
- ½ cup sour cream or plain full-fat Greek yogurt
- 1 Tbsp. tahini
- 1 Tbsp. fresh lemon juice

Instructions

2. Preheat oven to 450°F.

3. Place garlic cloves in a piece of a foil and drizzle with 1 tsp. olive oil. Wrap the garlic in the foil and place in the oven once it preheats. Continue roasting garlic while you prepare the potatoes.

4. Place the potatoes in a large pot, and cover them with one inch of cold water. Add 2 teaspoons salt and bring to a boil. Once the water is boiling, set the timer for 15 minutes.

5. At this point, the potatoes should be just past fork-tender. Drain potatoes.

6. In a large bowl, combine remaining ¼ cup olive oil, rosemary, sumac, remaining ½ tsp. salt, and black pepper. Add hot potatoes to mixture and let sit for 15 minutes, tossing occasionally.

7. Arrange potatoes on a baking sheet, making sure to leave about 2 inches of space in between each one.

8. Use the bottom of a measuring cup or a potato masher to gently "smash" each potato down until it is around ½-inch thick. Brush any of the remaining oil mixture from the bowl over the potatoes.

9. Roast potatoes for 20 to 25 minutes. Broil for the final 2 to 3 minutes for extra crispiness. *During the final 10 minutes of roasting, remove garlic from oven.

10. Remove garlic from peels and place on a cutting board. Use the prongs of a fork to throughly mash garlic into a paste. Add to a bowl along with sour cream, tahini, and lemon juice; mix well.

11. Transfer smashed potatoes to a serving platter and serve alongside dip. (I like to drizzle a little extra olive oil over the dip before serving, along with a grind of cracked black pepper.)